This Book Belongs To:

Emergency Contacts

Shot Location

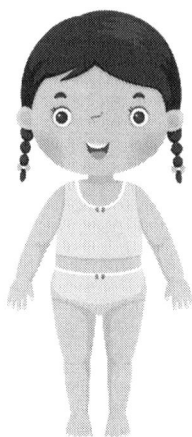

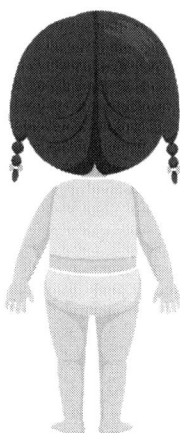

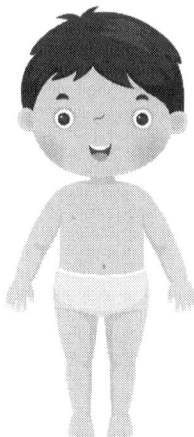

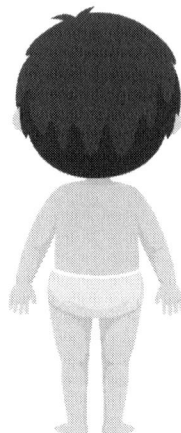

Notes

	Time	Blood Sugar	Carbs	Insulin	Notes
Breakfast					
Snack					
Lunch					
Snack					
Dinner					
Bedtime					
Night					

Shot Location

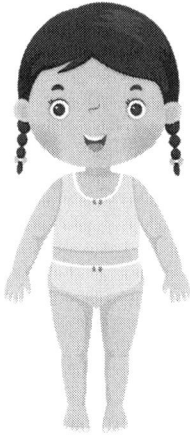

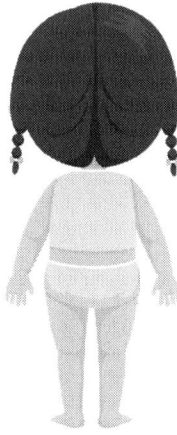

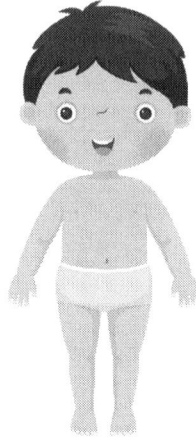

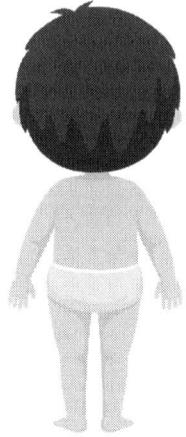

Notes

	Time	Blood Sugar	Carbs	Insulin	Notes
Breakfast					
Snack					
Lunch					
Snack					
Dinner					
Bedtime					
Night					

Shot Location

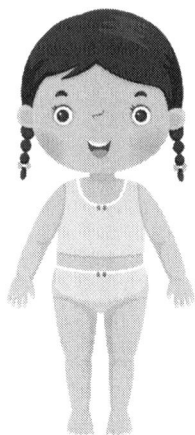

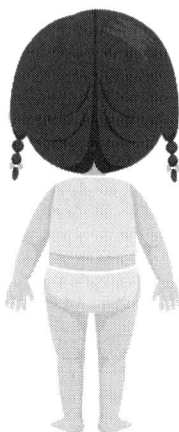

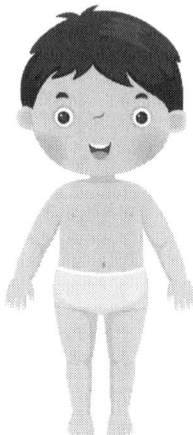

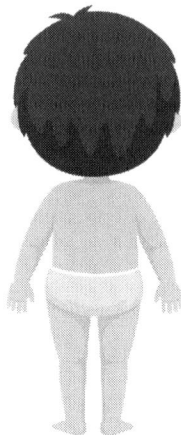

Notes

	Time	Blood Sugar	Carbs	Insulin	Notes
Breakfast					
Snack					
Lunch					
Snack					
Dinner					
Bedtime					
Night					

Shot Location

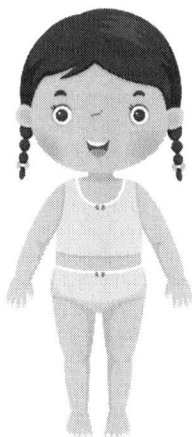

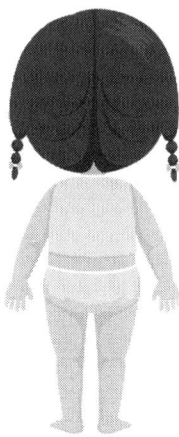

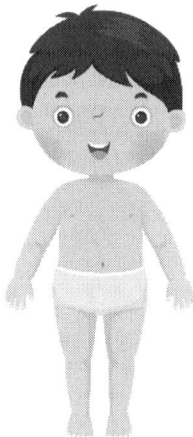

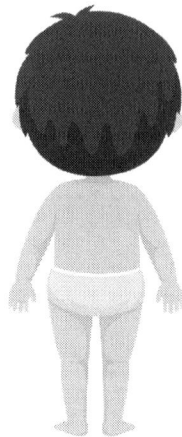

Notes

	Time	Blood Sugar	Carbs	Insulin	Notes
Breakfast					
Snack					
Lunch					
Snack					
Dinner					
Bedtime					
Night					

Shot Location

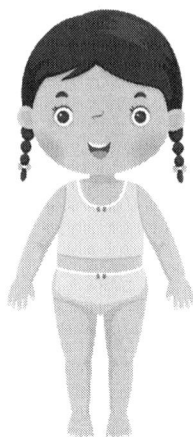

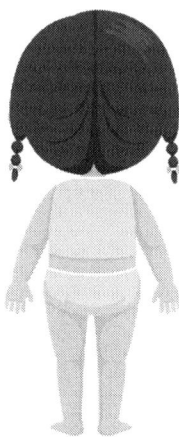

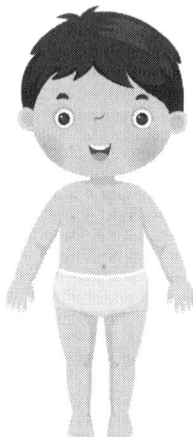

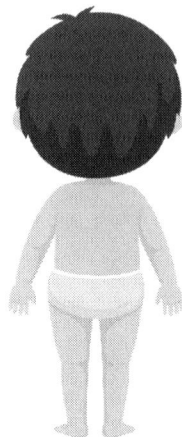

Notes

	Time	Blood Sugar	Carbs	Insulin	Notes
Breakfast					
Snack					
Lunch					
Snack					
Dinner					
Bedtime					
Night					

Shot Location

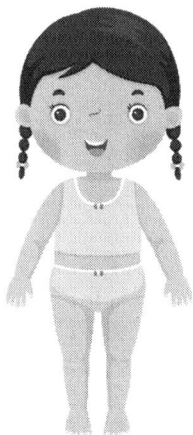

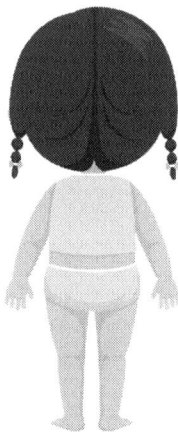

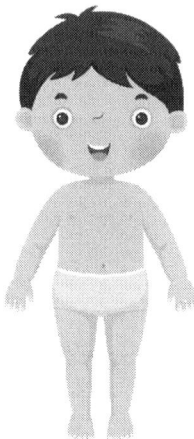

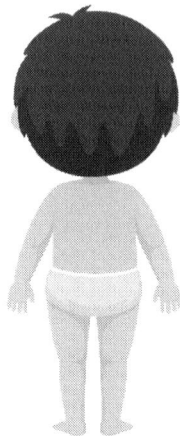

Notes

	Time	Blood Sugar	Carbs	Insulin	Notes
Breakfast					
Snack					
Lunch					
Snack					
Dinner					
Bedtime					
Night					

Shot Location

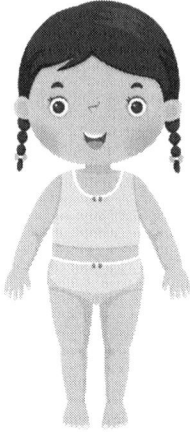

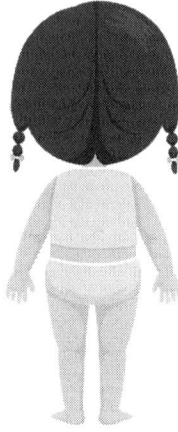

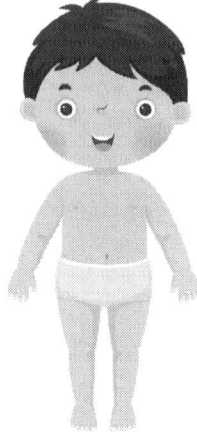

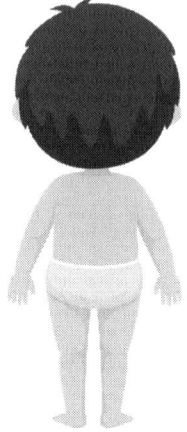

Notes

	Time	Blood Sugar	Carbs	Insulin	Notes
Breakfast					
Snack					
Lunch					
Snack					
Dinner					
Bedtime					
Night					

Shot Location

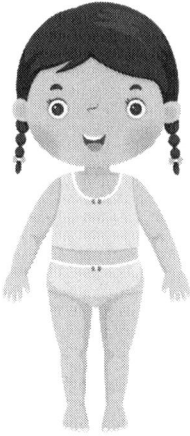

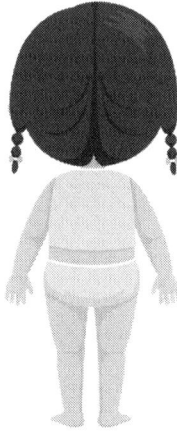

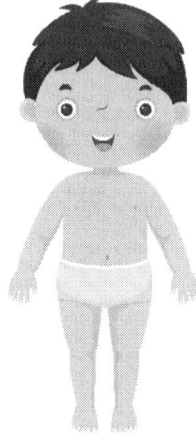

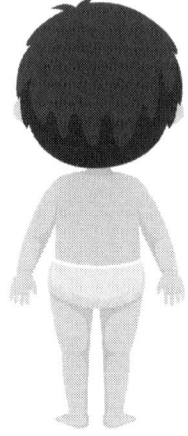

Notes

	Time	Blood Sugar	Carbs	Insulin	Notes
Breakfast					
Snack					
Lunch					
Snack					
Dinner					
Bedtime					
Night					

Shot Location

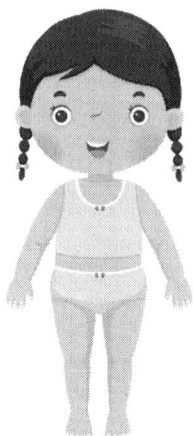

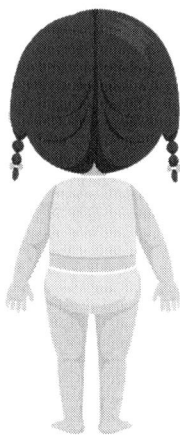

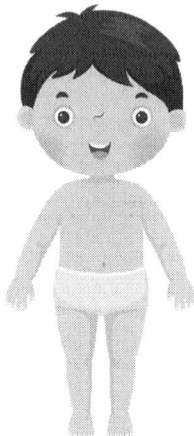

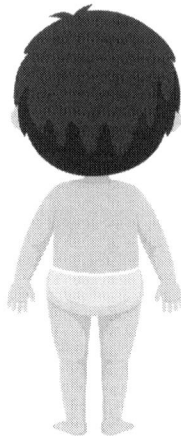

Notes

	Time	Blood Sugar	Carbs	Insulin	Notes
Breakfast					
Snack					
Lunch					
Snack					
Dinner					
Bedtime					
Night					

Shot Location

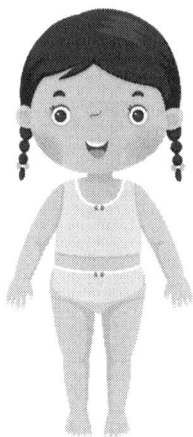

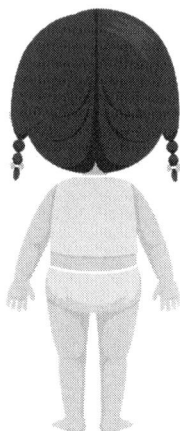

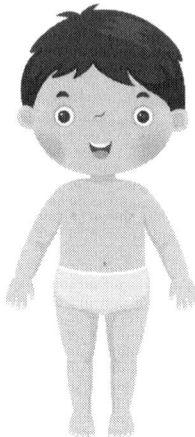

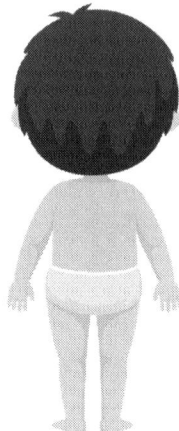

Notes

	Time	Blood Sugar	Carbs	Insulin	Notes
Breakfast					
Snack					
Lunch					
Snack					
Dinner					
Bedtime					
Night					

Shot Location

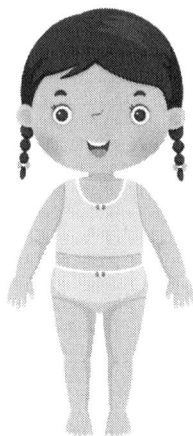

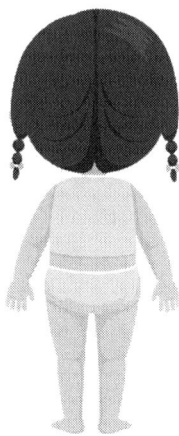

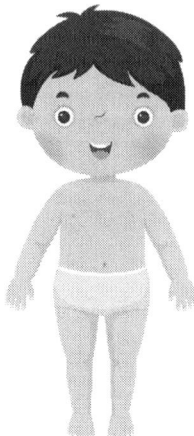

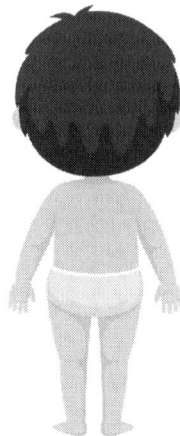

Notes

	Time	Blood Sugar	Carbs	Insulin	Notes
Breakfast					
Snack					
Lunch					
Snack					
Dinner					
Bedtime					
Night					

Shot Location

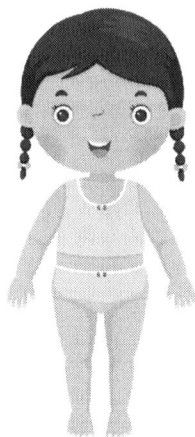

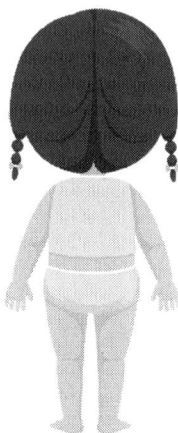

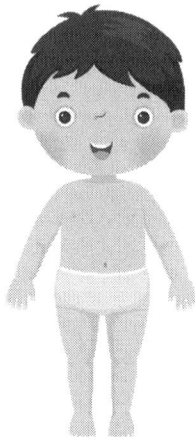

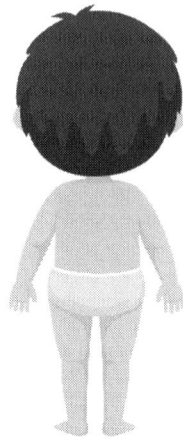

Notes

	Time	Blood Sugar	Carbs	Insulin	Notes
Breakfast					
Snack					
Lunch					
Snack					
Dinner					
Bedtime					
Night					

Shot Location

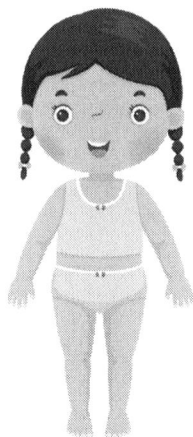

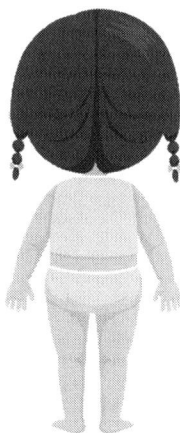

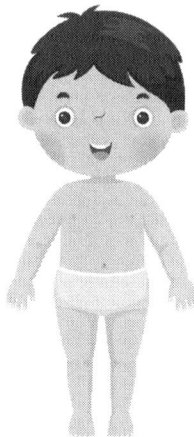

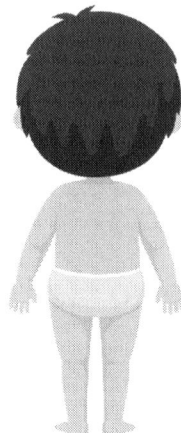

Notes

	Time	Blood Sugar	Carbs	Insulin	Notes
Breakfast					
Snack					
Lunch					
Snack					
Dinner					
Bedtime					
Night					

Shot Location

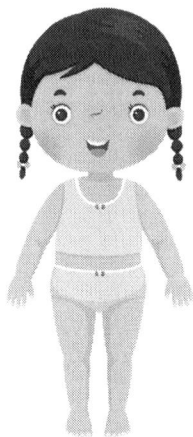

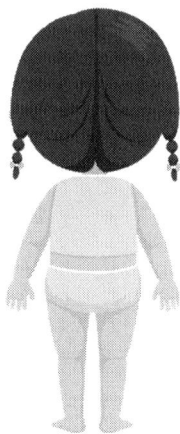

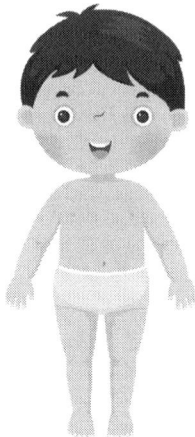

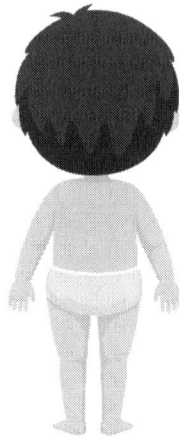

Notes

	Time	Blood Sugar	Carbs	Insulin	Notes
Breakfast					
Snack					
Lunch					
Snack					
Dinner					
Bedtime					
Night					

Shot Location

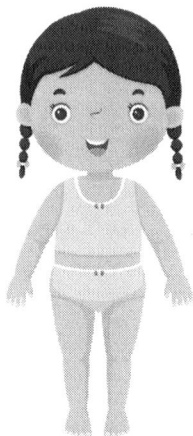

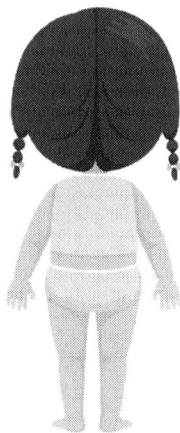

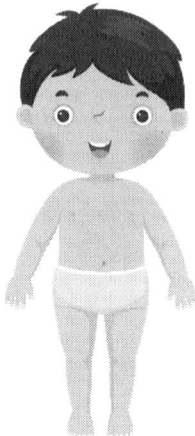

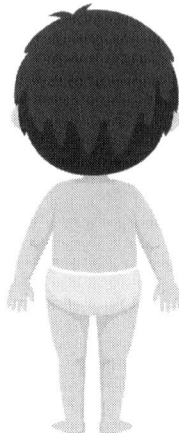

Notes

	Time	Blood Sugar	Carbs	Insulin	Notes
Breakfast					
Snack					
Lunch					
Snack					
Dinner					
Bedtime					
Night					

Shot Location

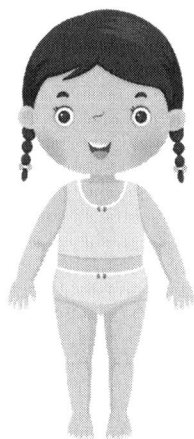

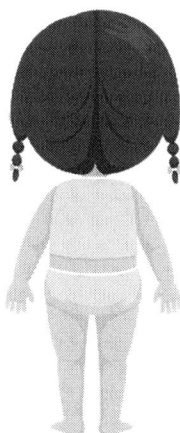

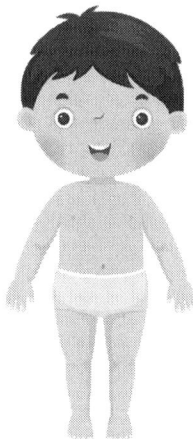

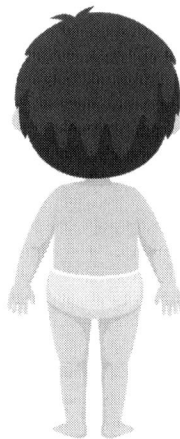

Notes

	Time	Blood Sugar	Carbs	Insulin	Notes
Breakfast					
Snack					
Lunch					
Snack					
Dinner					
Bedtime					
Night					

Shot Location

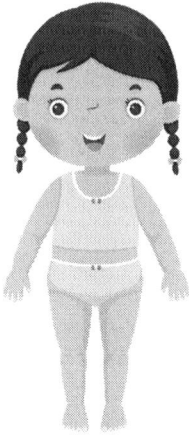

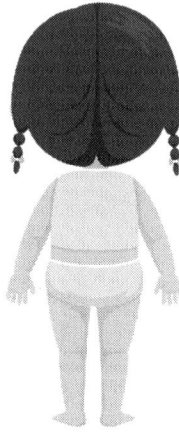

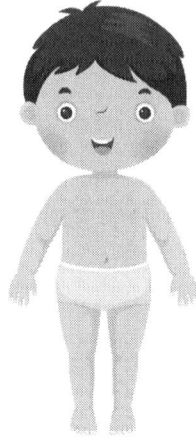

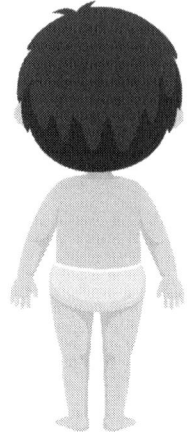

Notes

M T W TH F S SU

Date: /   /

	Time	Blood Sugar	Carbs	Insulin	Notes
Breakfast					
Snack					
Lunch					
Snack					
Dinner					
Bedtime					
Night					

Shot Location

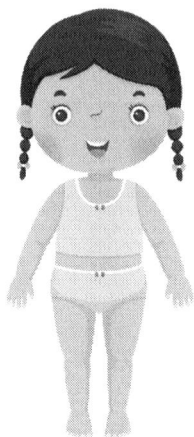

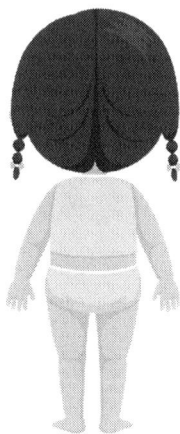

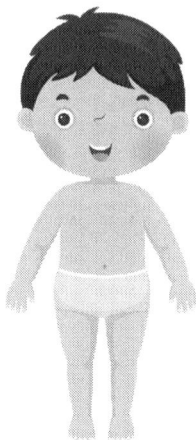

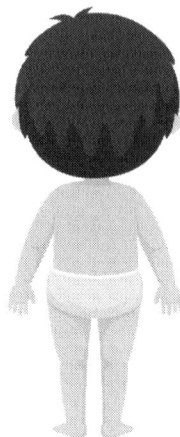

Notes

	Time	Blood Sugar	Carbs	Insulin	Notes
Breakfast					
Snack					
Lunch					
Snack					
Dinner					
Bedtime					
Night					

Shot Location

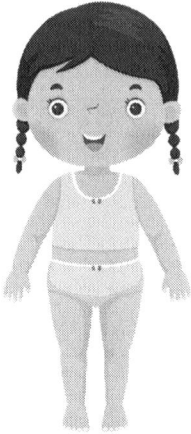

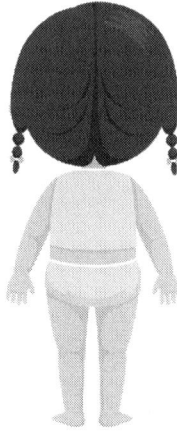

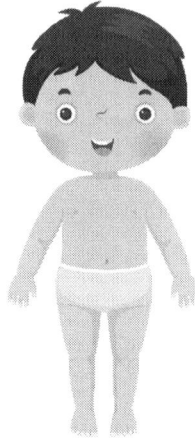

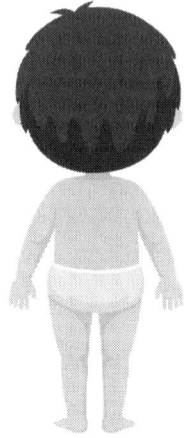

Notes

	Time	Blood Sugar	Carbs	Insulin	Notes
Breakfast					
Snack					
Lunch					
Snack					
Dinner					
Bedtime					
Night					

Shot Location

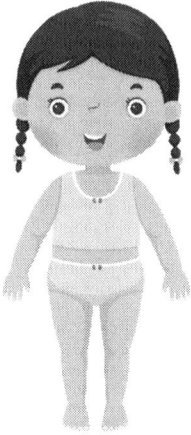

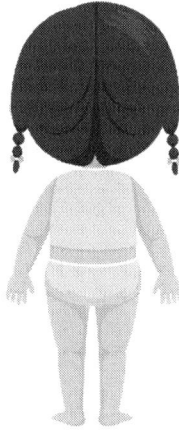

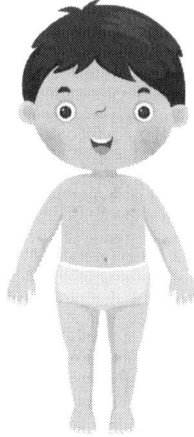

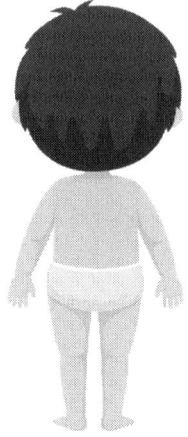

Notes

	Time	Blood Sugar	Carbs	Insulin	Notes
Breakfast					
Snack					
Lunch					
Snack					
Dinner					
Bedtime					
Night					

Shot Location

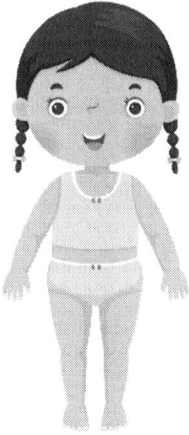

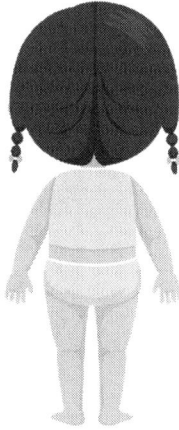

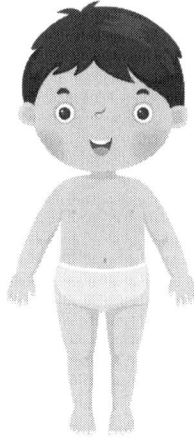

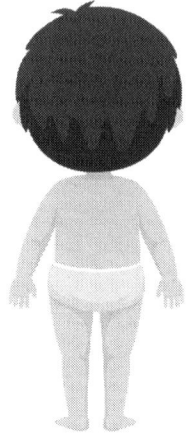

Notes

	Time	Blood Sugar	Carbs	Insulin	Notes
Breakfast					
Snack					
Lunch					
Snack					
Dinner					
Bedtime					
Night					

Shot Location

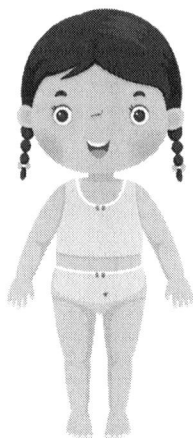

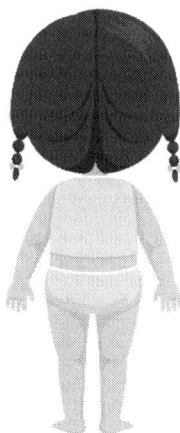

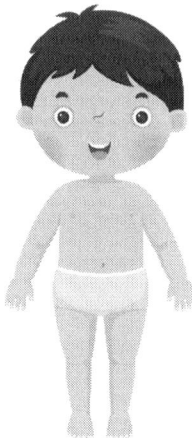

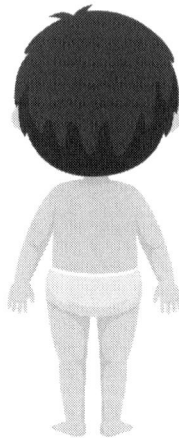

Notes

	Time	Blood Sugar	Carbs	Insulin	Notes
Breakfast					
Snack					
Lunch					
Snack					
Dinner					
Bedtime					
Night					

Shot Location

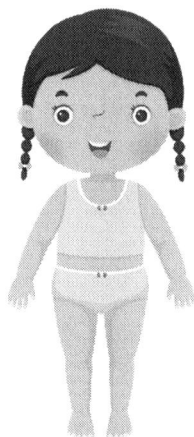

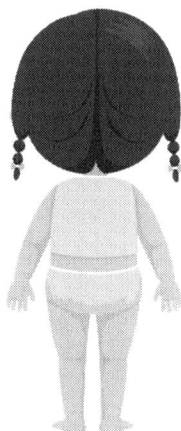

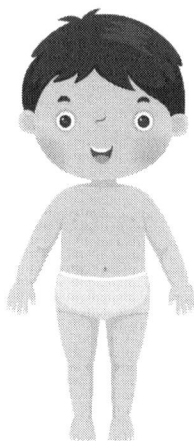

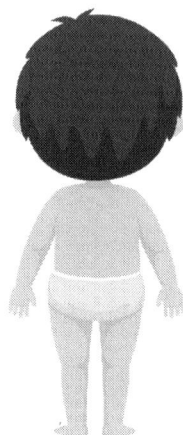

Notes

	Time	Blood Sugar	Carbs	Insulin	Notes
Breakfast					
Snack					
Lunch					
Snack					
Dinner					
Bedtime					
Night					

Shot Location

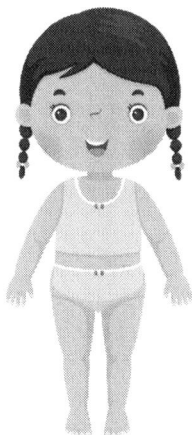

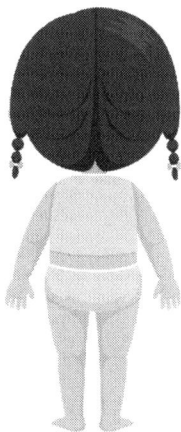

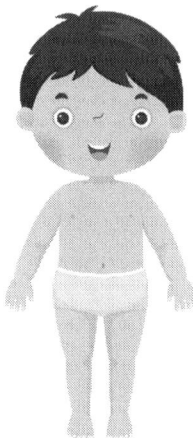

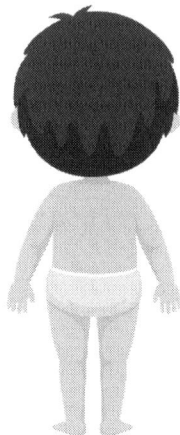

Notes

	Time	Blood Sugar	Carbs	Insulin	Notes
Breakfast					
Snack					
Lunch					
Snack					
Dinner					
Bedtime					
Night					

Shot Location

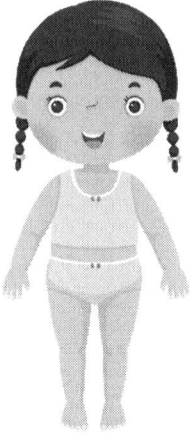

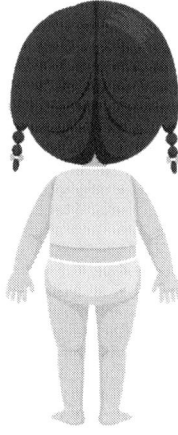

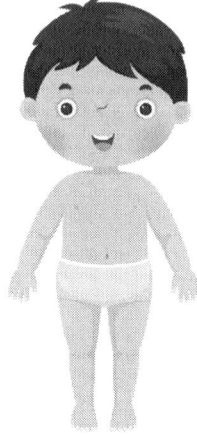

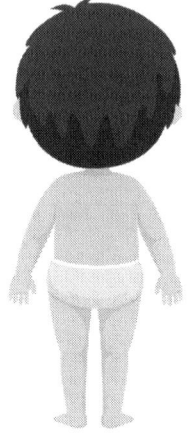

Notes

	Time	Blood Sugar	Carbs	Insulin	Notes
Breakfast					
Snack					
Lunch					
Snack					
Dinner					
Bedtime					
Night					

Shot Location

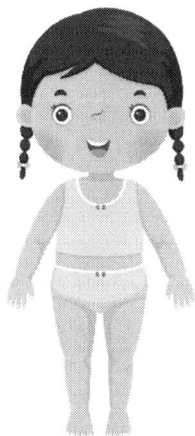

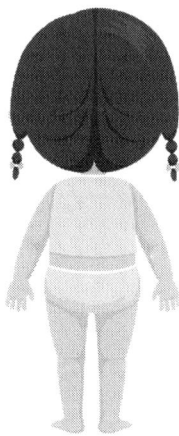

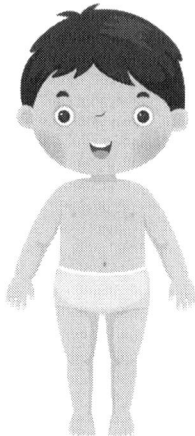

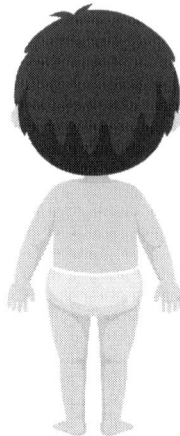

Notes

	Time	Blood Sugar	Carbs	Insulin	Notes
Breakfast					
Snack					
Lunch					
Snack					
Dinner					
Bedtime					
Night					

Shot Location

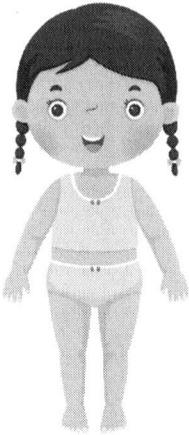

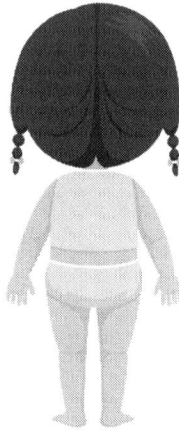

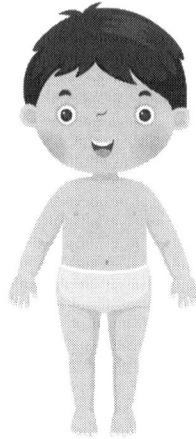

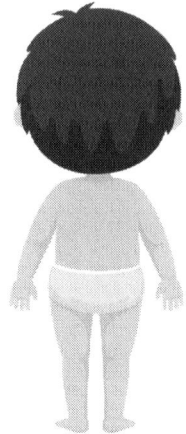

Notes

	Time	Blood Sugar	Carbs	Insulin	Notes
Breakfast					
Snack					
Lunch					
Snack					
Dinner					
Bedtime					
Night					

Shot Location

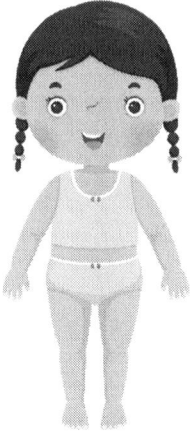

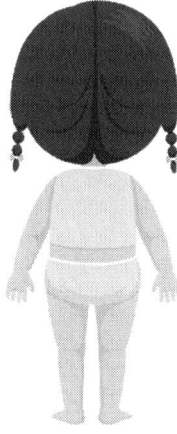

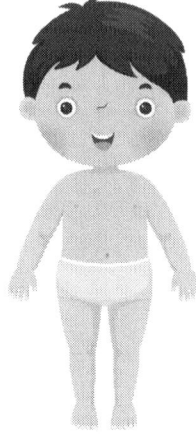

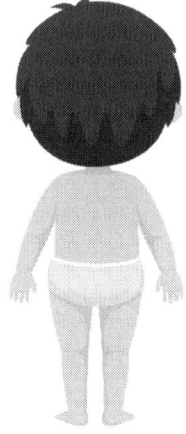

Notes

	Time	Blood Sugar	Carbs	Insulin	Notes
Breakfast					
Snack					
Lunch					
Snack					
Dinner					
Bedtime					
Night					

Shot Location

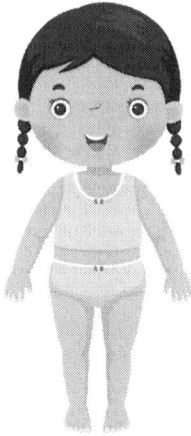

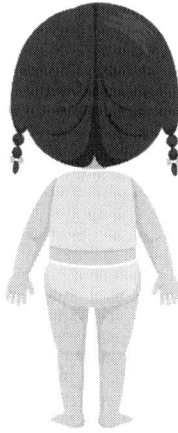

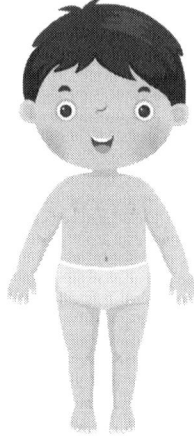

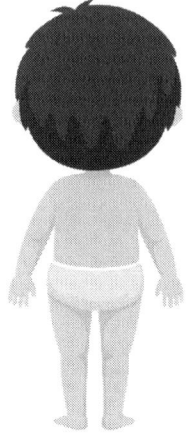

Notes

	Time	Blood Sugar	Carbs	Insulin	Notes
Breakfast					
Snack					
Lunch					
Snack					
Dinner					
Bedtime					
Night					

Shot Location

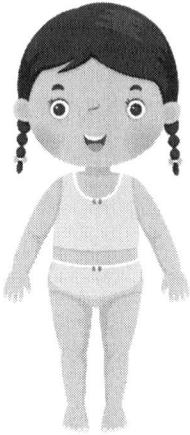

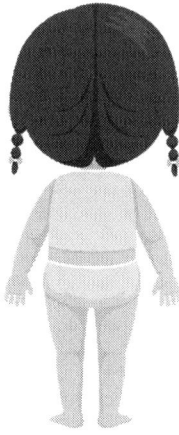

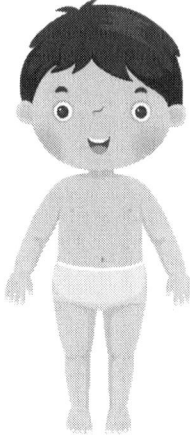

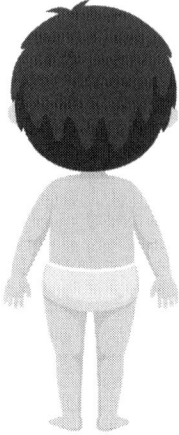

Notes

	Time	Blood Sugar	Carbs	Insulin	Notes
Breakfast					
Snack					
Lunch					
Snack					
Dinner					
Bedtime					
Night					

Shot Location

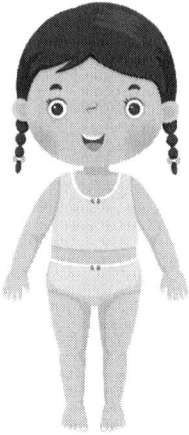

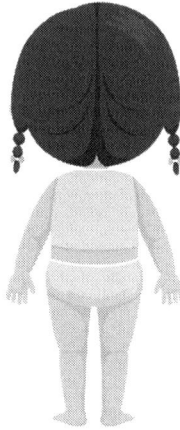

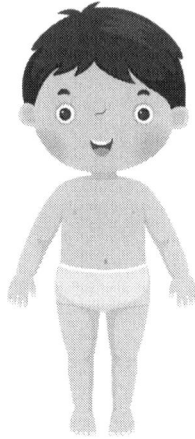

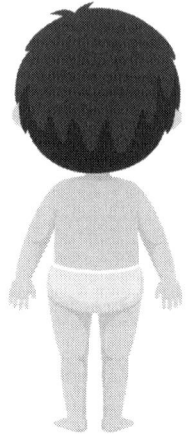

Notes

	Time	Blood Sugar	Carbs	Insulin	Notes
Breakfast					
Snack					
Lunch					
Snack					
Dinner					
Bedtime					
Night					

Shot Location

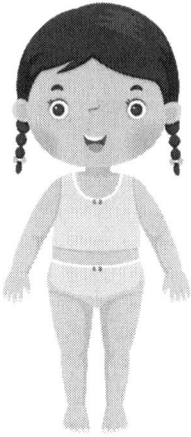

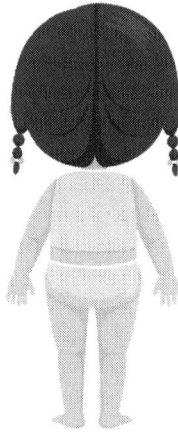

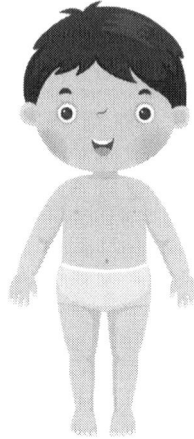

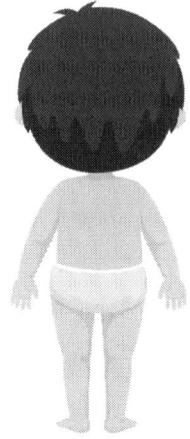

Notes

	Time	Blood Sugar	Carbs	Insulin	Notes
Breakfast					
Snack					
Lunch					
Snack					
Dinner					
Bedtime					
Night					

Shot Location

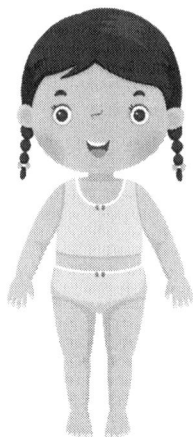

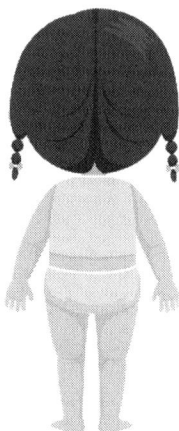

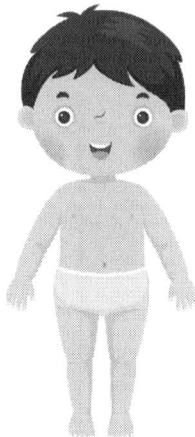

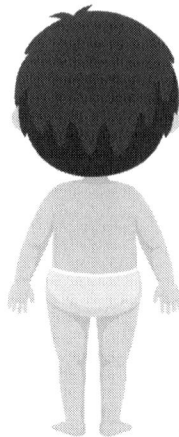

Notes

	Time	Blood Sugar	Carbs	Insulin	Notes
Breakfast					
Snack					
Lunch					
Snack					
Dinner					
Bedtime					
Night					

Shot Location

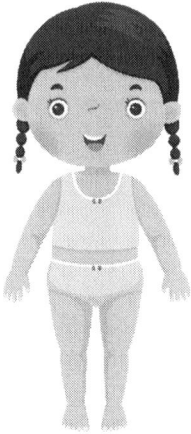

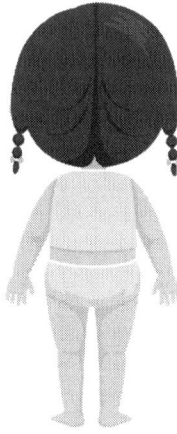

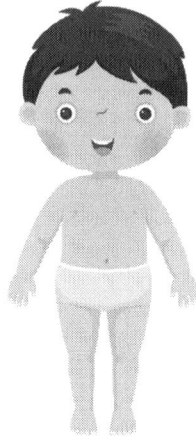

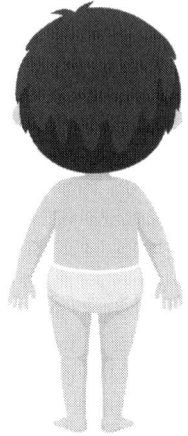

Notes

	Time	Blood Sugar	Carbs	Insulin	Notes
Breakfast					
Snack					
Lunch					
Snack					
Dinner					
Bedtime					
Night					

Shot Location

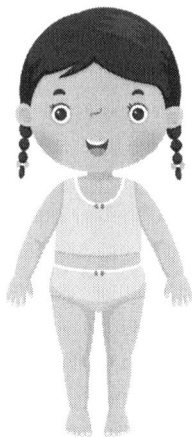

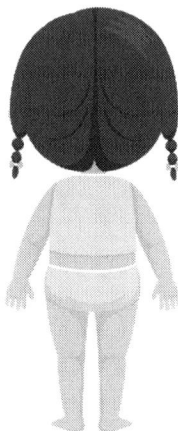

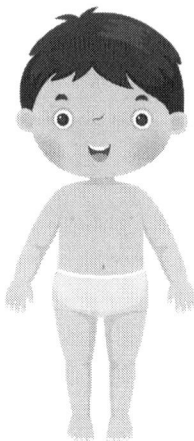

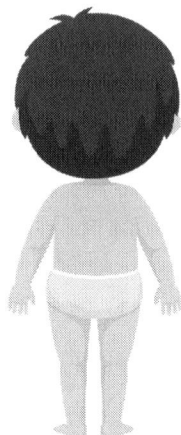

Notes

	Time	Blood Sugar	Carbs	Insulin	Notes
Breakfast					
Snack					
Lunch					
Snack					
Dinner					
Bedtime					
Night					

Shot Location

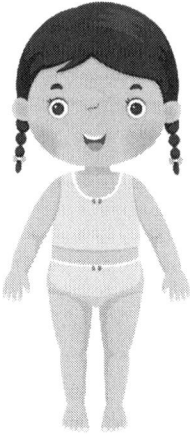

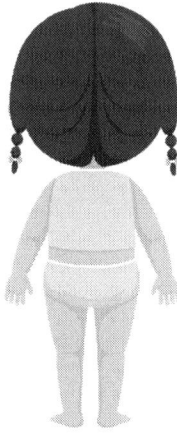

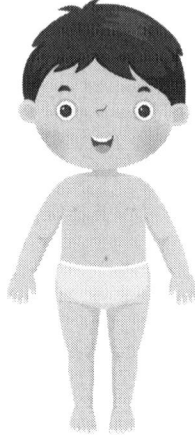

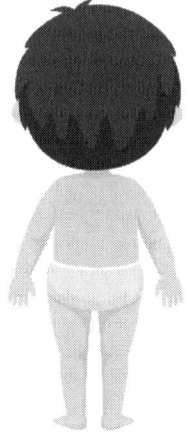

Notes

	Time	Blood Sugar	Carbs	Insulin	Notes
Breakfast					
Snack					
Lunch					
Snack					
Dinner					
Bedtime					
Night					

Shot Location

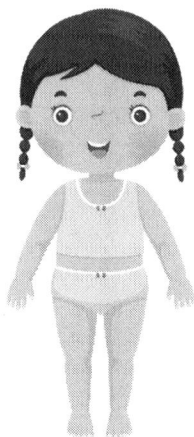

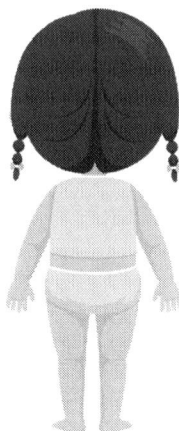

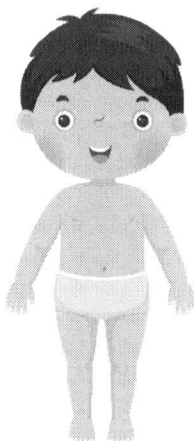

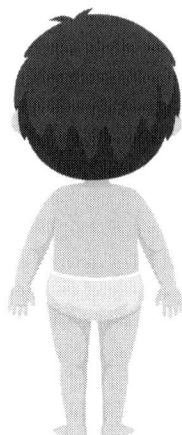

Notes

	Time	Blood Sugar	Carbs	Insulin	Notes
Breakfast					
Snack					
Lunch					
Snack					
Dinner					
Bedtime					
Night					

Shot Location

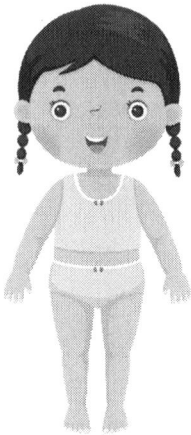

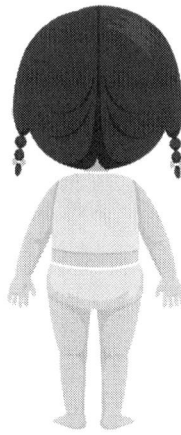

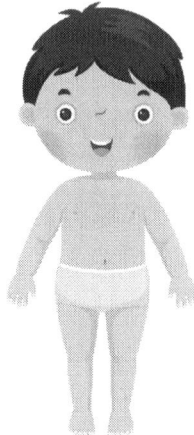

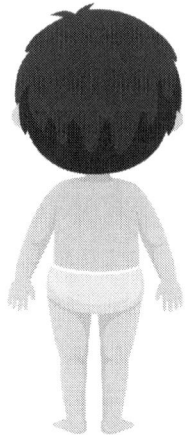

Notes

	Time	Blood Sugar	Carbs	Insulin	Notes
Breakfast					
Snack					
Lunch					
Snack					
Dinner					
Bedtime					
Night					

Shot Location

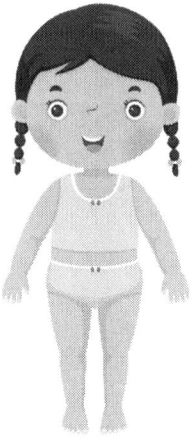

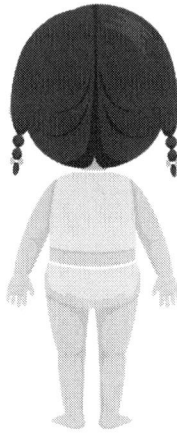

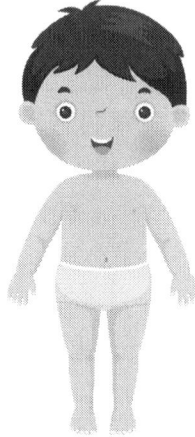

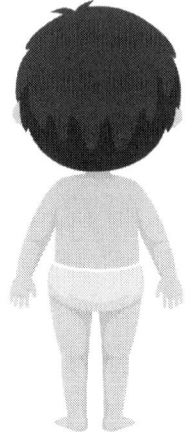

Notes

	Time	Blood Sugar	Carbs	Insulin	Notes
Breakfast					
Snack					
Lunch					
Snack					
Dinner					
Bedtime					
Night					

Shot Location

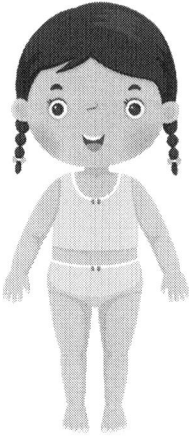

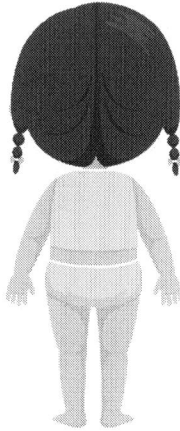

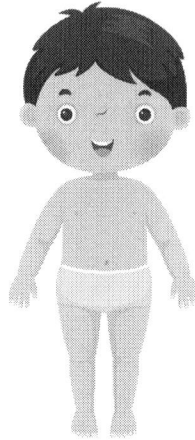

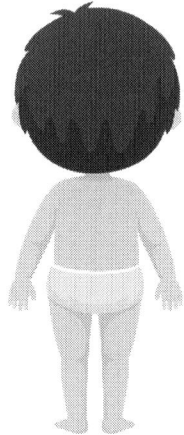

Notes

	Time	Blood Sugar	Carbs	Insulin	Notes
Breakfast					
Snack					
Lunch					
Snack					
Dinner					
Bedtime					
Night					

Shot Location

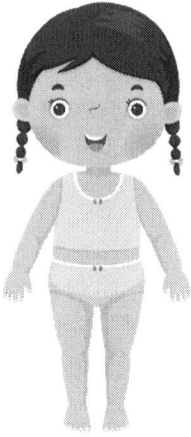

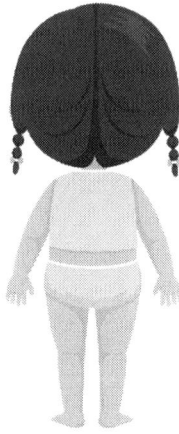

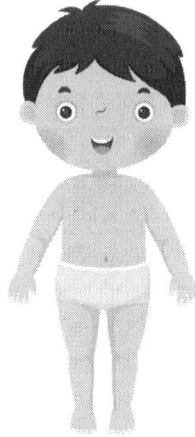

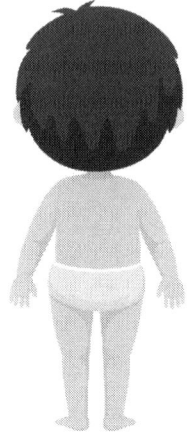

Notes

	Time	Blood Sugar	Carbs	Insulin	Notes
Breakfast					
Snack					
Lunch					
Snack					
Dinner					
Bedtime					
Night					

Shot Location

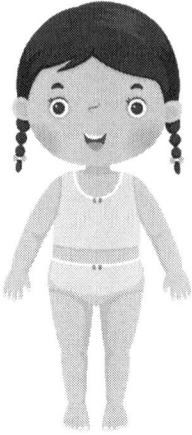

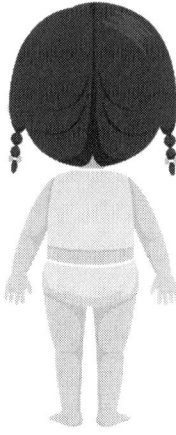

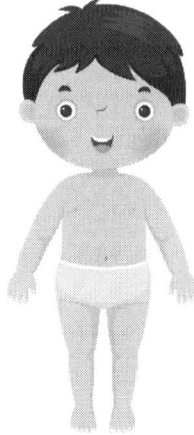

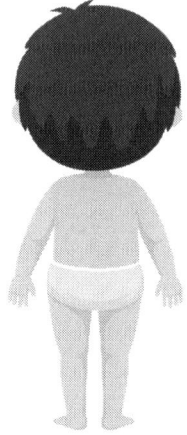

Notes

	Time	Blood Sugar	Carbs	Insulin	Notes
Breakfast					
Snack					
Lunch					
Snack					
Dinner					
Bedtime					
Night					

Shot Location

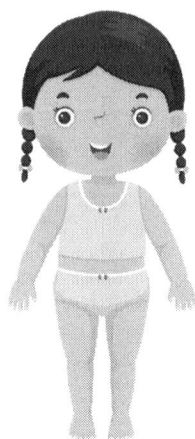

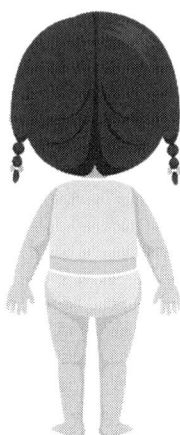

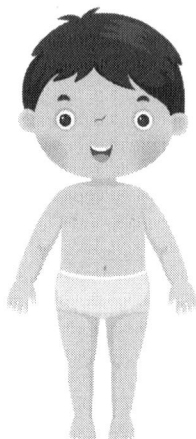

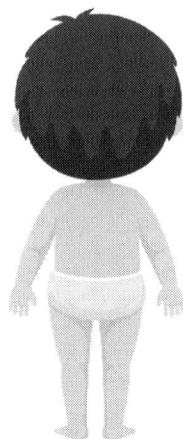

Notes

	Time	Blood Sugar	Carbs	Insulin	Notes
Breakfast					
Snack					
Lunch					
Snack					
Dinner					
Bedtime					
Night					

Shot Location

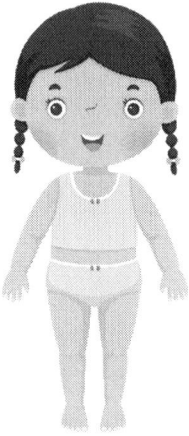

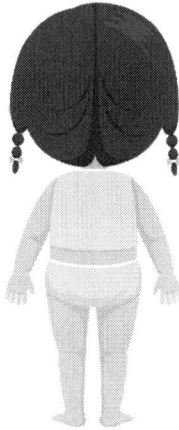

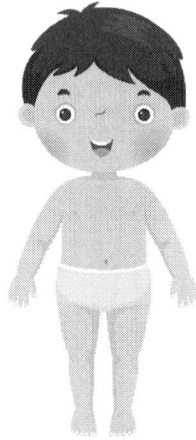

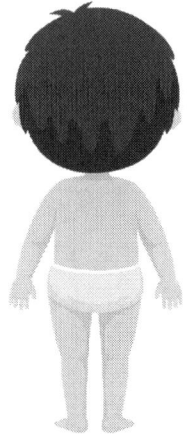

Notes

	Time	Blood Sugar	Carbs	Insulin	Notes
Breakfast					
Snack					
Lunch					
Snack					
Dinner					
Bedtime					
Night					

Shot Location

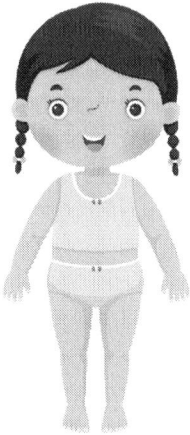

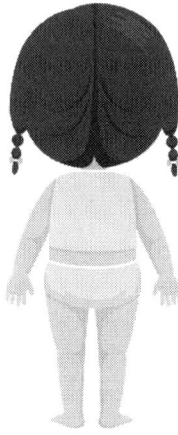

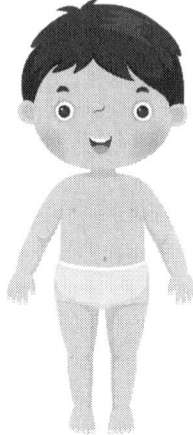

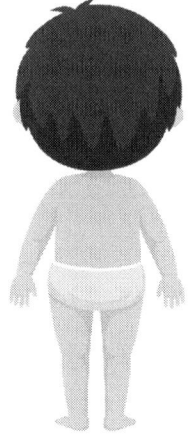

Notes

	Time	Blood Sugar	Carbs	Insulin	Notes
Breakfast					
Snack					
Lunch					
Snack					
Dinner					
Bedtime					
Night					

Shot Location

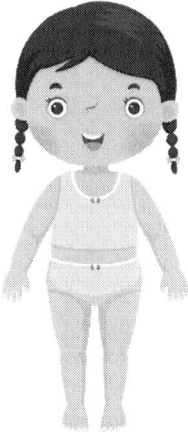

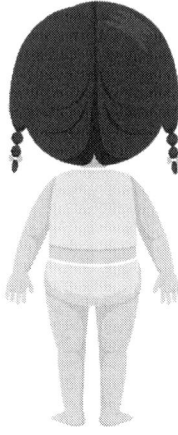

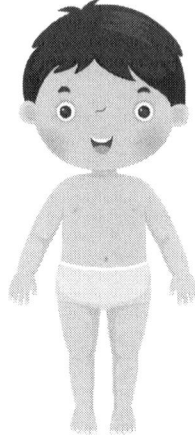

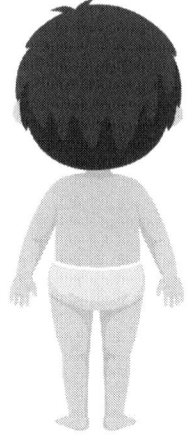

Notes

	Time	Blood Sugar	Carbs	Insulin	Notes
Breakfast					
Snack					
Lunch					
Snack					
Dinner					
Bedtime					
Night					

Shot Location

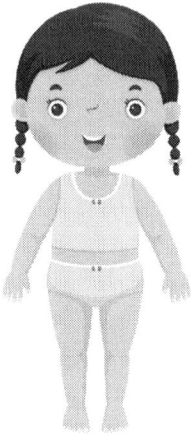

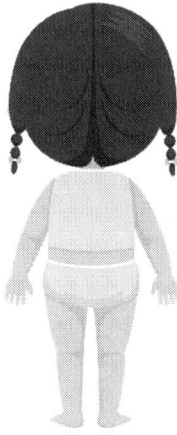

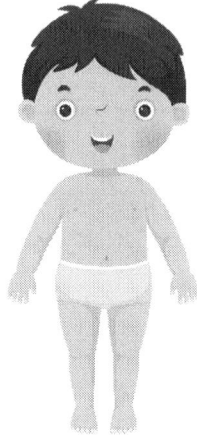

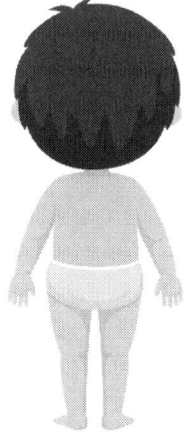

Notes

	Time	Blood Sugar	Carbs	Insulin	Notes
Breakfast					
Snack					
Lunch					
Snack					
Dinner					
Bedtime					
Night					

Shot Location

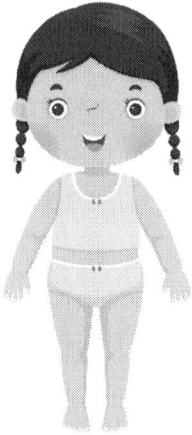

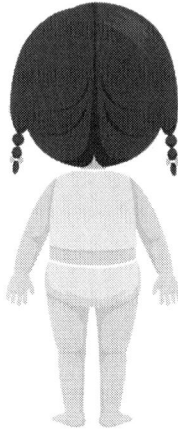

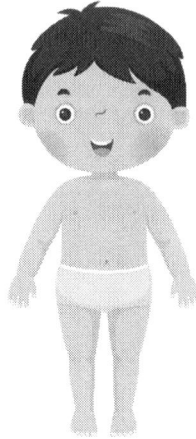

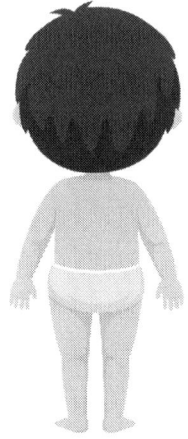

Notes

	Time	Blood Sugar	Carbs	Insulin	Notes
Breakfast					
Snack					
Lunch					
Snack					
Dinner					
Bedtime					
Night					

Shot Location

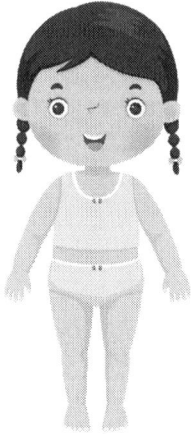

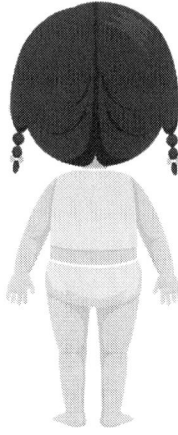

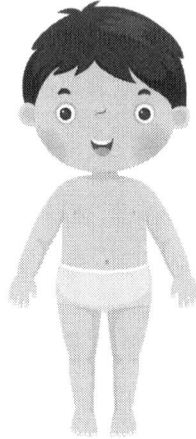

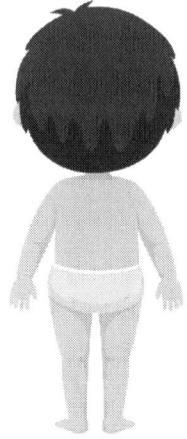

Notes

	Time	Blood Sugar	Carbs	Insulin	Notes
Breakfast					
Snack					
Lunch					
Snack					
Dinner					
Bedtime					
Night					

Shot Location

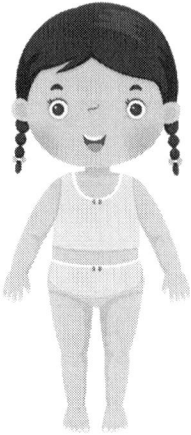

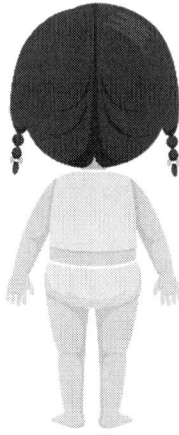

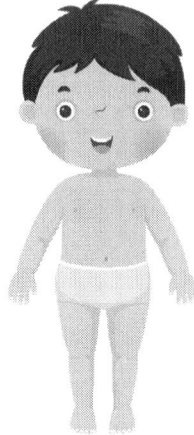

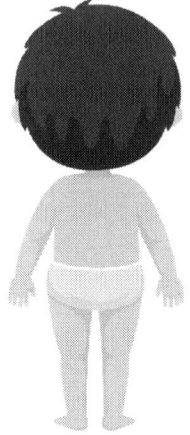

Notes

	Time	Blood Sugar	Carbs	Insulin	Notes
Breakfast					
Snack					
Lunch					
Snack					
Dinner					
Bedtime					
Night					

Shot Location

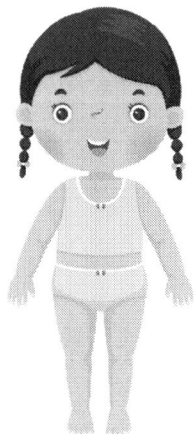

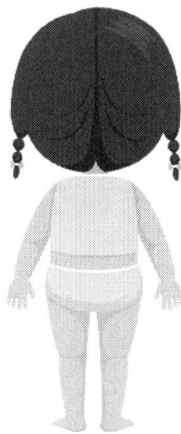

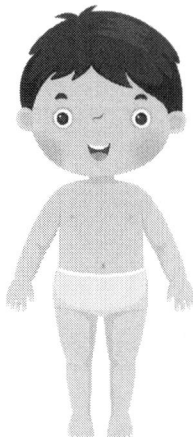

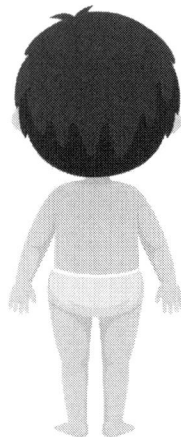

Notes

	Time	Blood Sugar	Carbs	Insulin	Notes
Breakfast					
Snack					
Lunch					
Snack					
Dinner					
Bedtime					
Night					

Shot Location

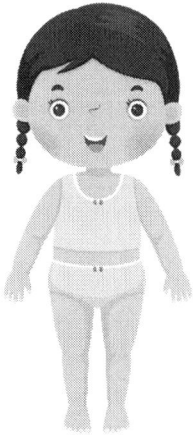

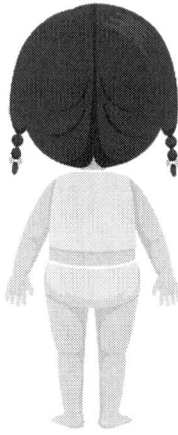

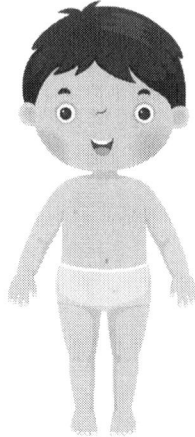

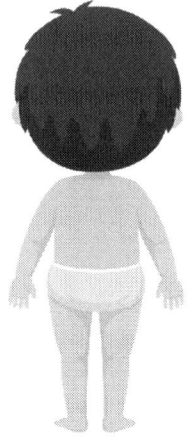

Notes

	Time	Blood Sugar	Carbs	Insulin	Notes
Breakfast					
Snack					
Lunch					
Snack					
Dinner					
Bedtime					
Night					

Shot Location

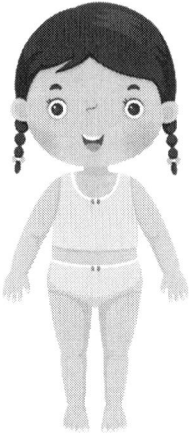

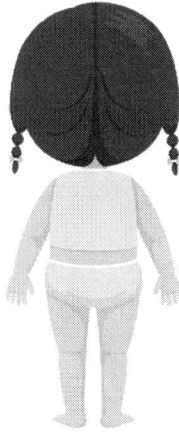

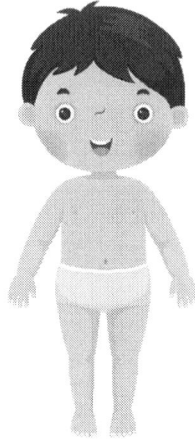

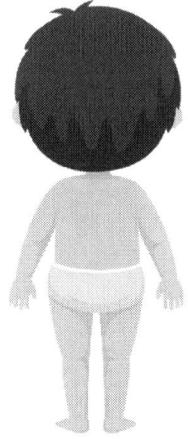

Notes

	Time	Blood Sugar	Carbs	Insulin	Notes
Breakfast					
Snack					
Lunch					
Snack					
Dinner					
Bedtime					
Night					

Shot Location

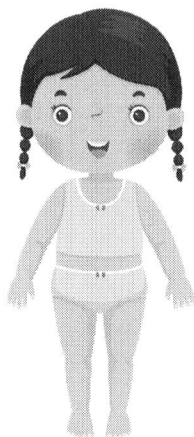

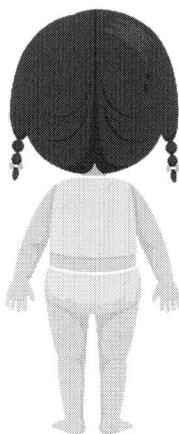

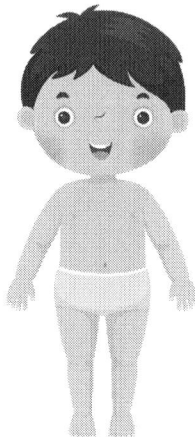

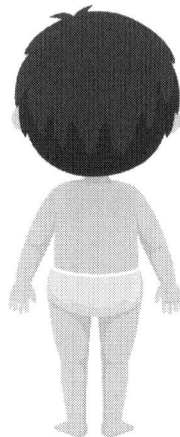

Notes

	Time	Blood Sugar	Carbs	Insulin	Notes
Breakfast					
Snack					
Lunch					
Snack					
Dinner					
Bedtime					
Night					

Shot Location

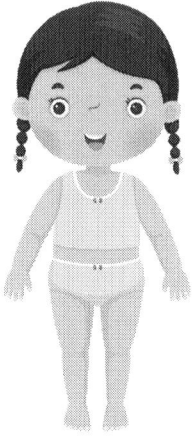

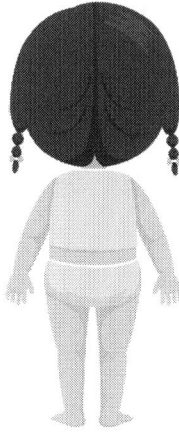

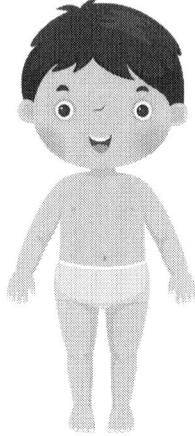

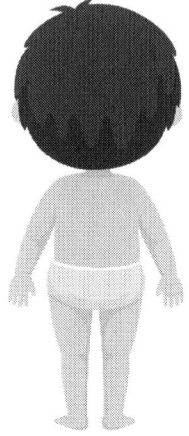

Notes

	Time	Blood Sugar	Carbs	Insulin	Notes
Breakfast					
Snack					
Lunch					
Snack					
Dinner					
Bedtime					
Night					

Shot Location

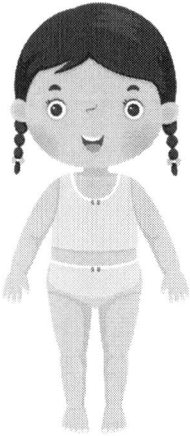

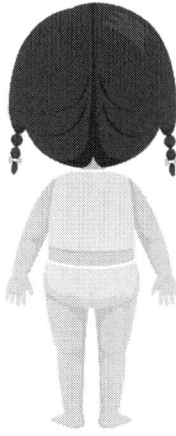

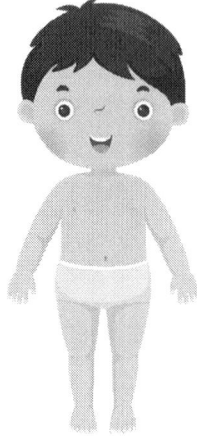

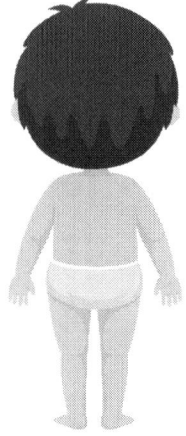

Notes

	Time	Blood Sugar	Carbs	Insulin	Notes
Breakfast					
Snack					
Lunch					
Snack					
Dinner					
Bedtime					
Night					

Shot Location

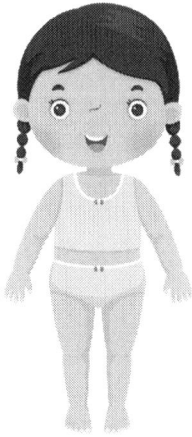

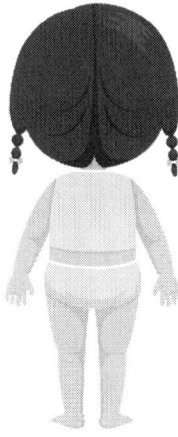

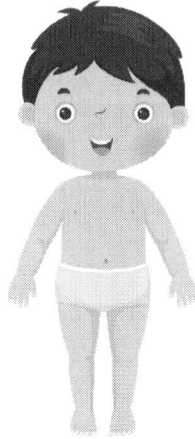

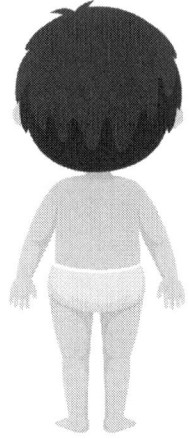

Notes

	Time	Blood Sugar	Carbs	Insulin	Notes
Breakfast					
Snack					
Lunch					
Snack					
Dinner					
Bedtime					
Night					

Shot Location

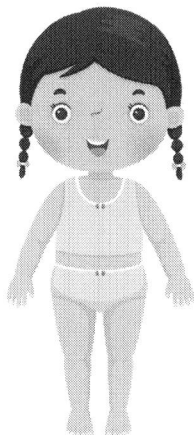

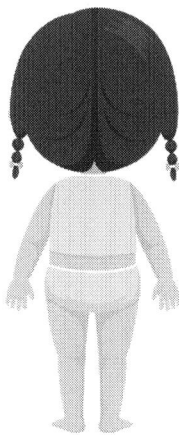

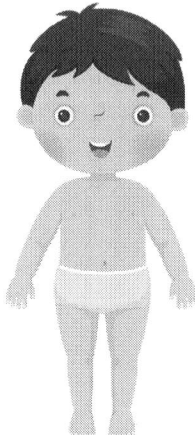

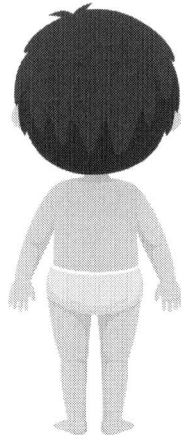

Notes

	Time	Blood Sugar	Carbs	Insulin	Notes
Breakfast					
Snack					
Lunch					
Snack					
Dinner					
Bedtime					
Night					

Shot Location

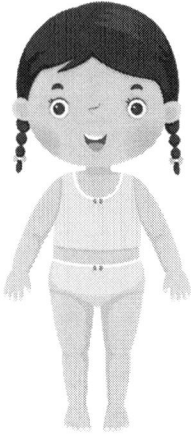

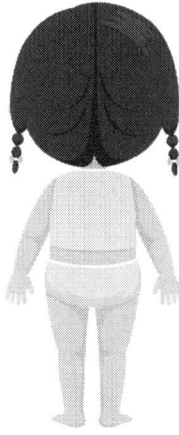

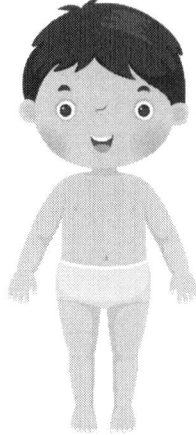

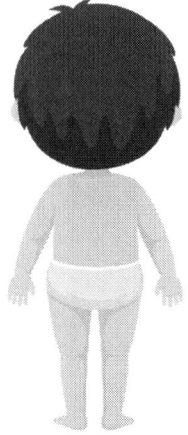

Notes

	Time	Blood Sugar	Carbs	Insulin	Notes
Breakfast					
Snack					
Lunch					
Snack					
Dinner					
Bedtime					
Night					

Shot Location

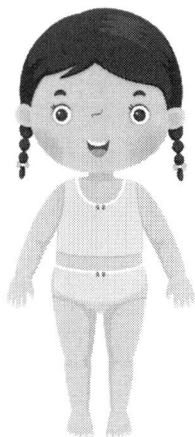

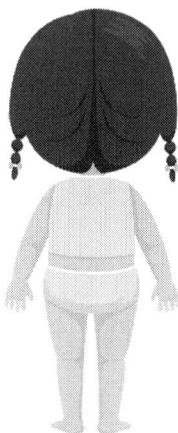

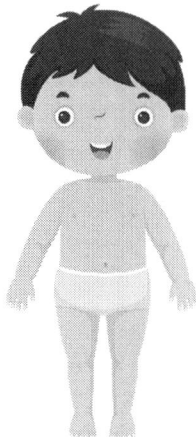

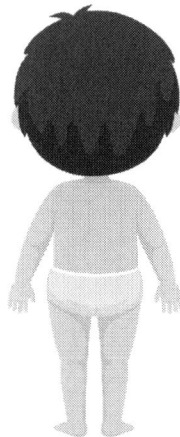

Notes

	Time	Blood Sugar	Carbs	Insulin	Notes
Breakfast					
Snack					
Lunch					
Snack					
Dinner					
Bedtime					
Night					

Shot Location

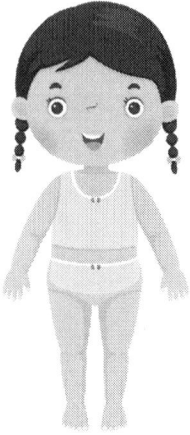

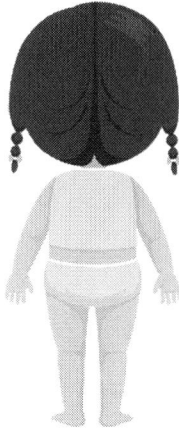

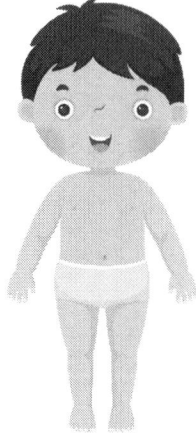

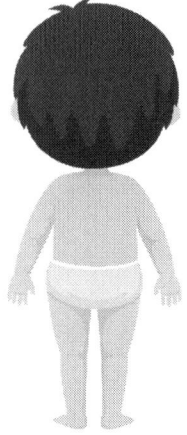

Notes

	Time	Blood Sugar	Carbs	Insulin	Notes
Breakfast					
Snack					
Lunch					
Snack					
Dinner					
Bedtime					
Night					

Shot Location

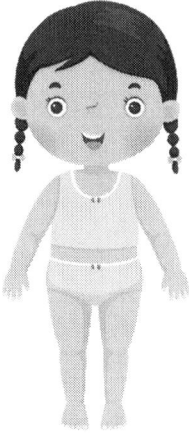

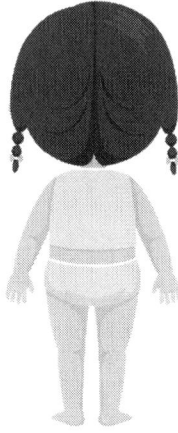

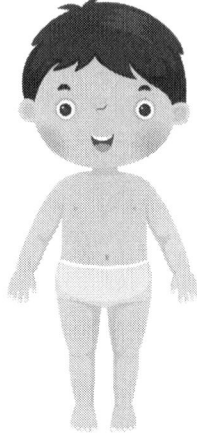

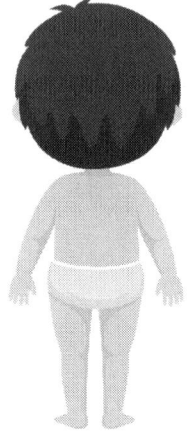

Notes

	Time	Blood Sugar	Carbs	Insulin	Notes
Breakfast					
Snack					
Lunch					
Snack					
Dinner					
Bedtime					
Night					

Shot Location

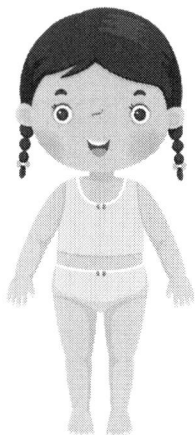

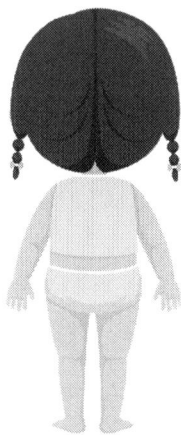

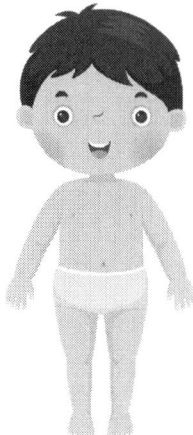

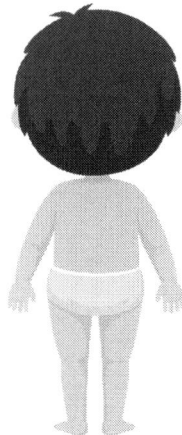

Notes

	Time	Blood Sugar	Carbs	Insulin	Notes
Breakfast					
Snack					
Lunch					
Snack					
Dinner					
Bedtime					
Night					

Shot Location

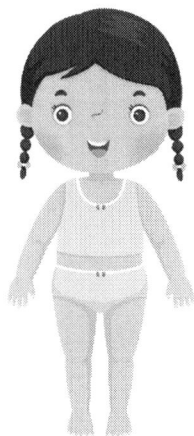

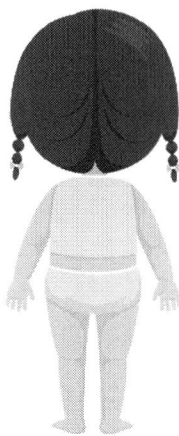

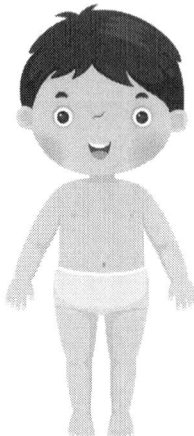

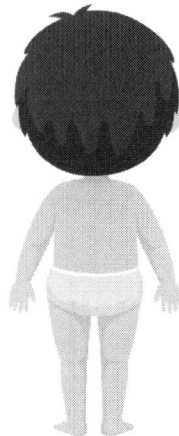

Notes

	Time	Blood Sugar	Carbs	Insulin	Notes
Breakfast					
Snack					
Lunch					
Snack					
Dinner					
Bedtime					
Night					

Shot Location

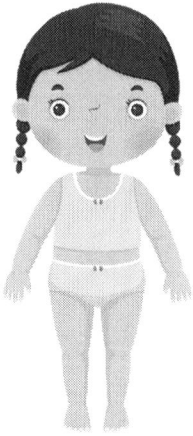

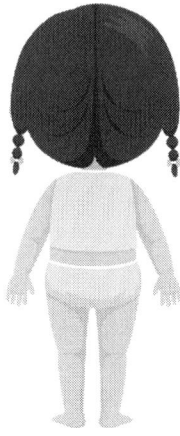

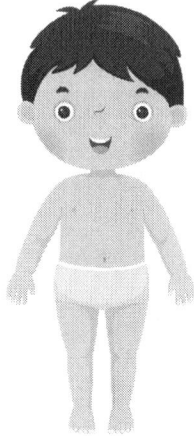

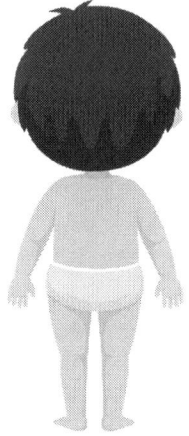

Notes

	Time	Blood Sugar	Carbs	Insulin	Notes
Breakfast					
Snack					
Lunch					
Snack					
Dinner					
Bedtime					
Night					

Shot Location

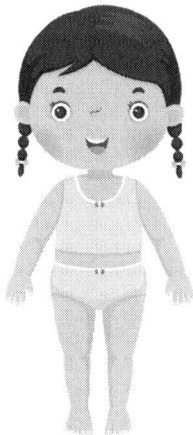

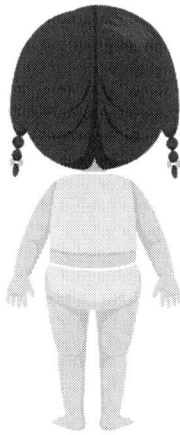

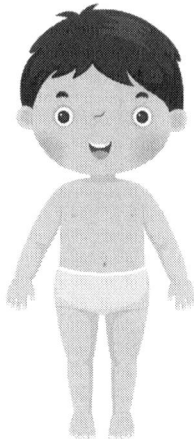

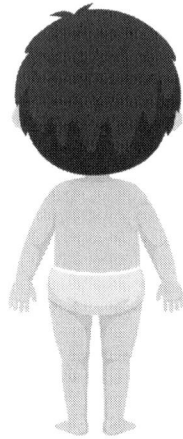

Notes

	Time	Blood Sugar	Carbs	Insulin	Notes
Breakfast					
Snack					
Lunch					
Snack					
Dinner					
Bedtime					
Night					

Shot Location

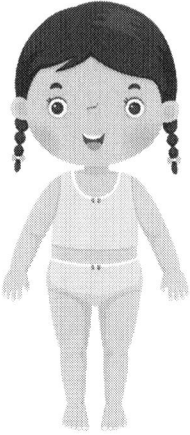

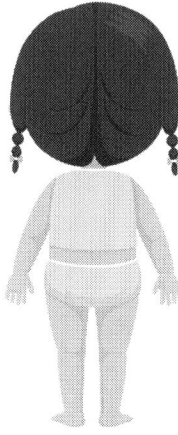

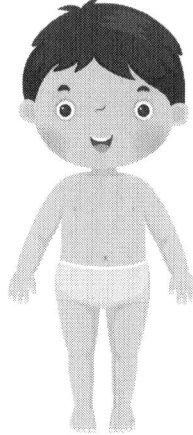

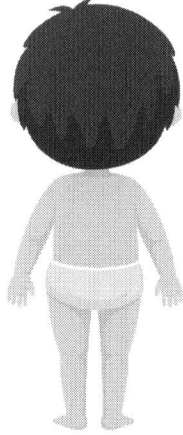

Notes

	Time	Blood Sugar	Carbs	Insulin	Notes
Breakfast					
Snack					
Lunch					
Snack					
Dinner					
Bedtime					
Night					

Shot Location

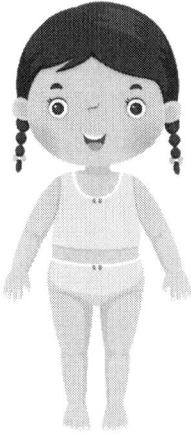

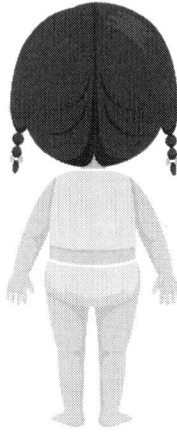

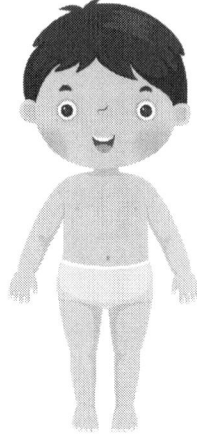

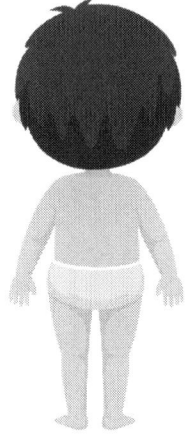

Notes

	Time	Blood Sugar	Carbs	Insulin	Notes
Breakfast					
Snack					
Lunch					
Snack					
Dinner					
Bedtime					
Night					

Shot Location

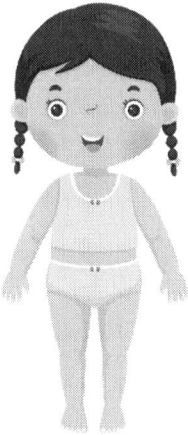

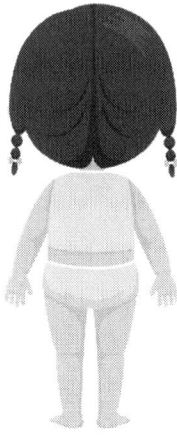

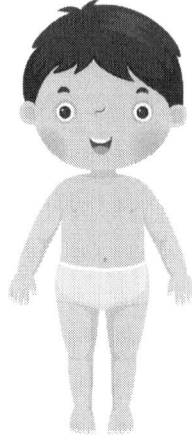

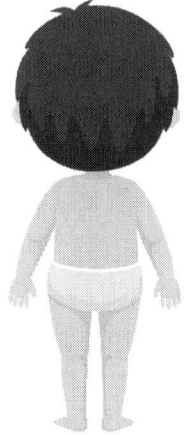

Notes

	Time	Blood Sugar	Carbs	Insulin	Notes
Breakfast					
Snack					
Lunch					
Snack					
Dinner					
Bedtime					
Night					

Shot Location

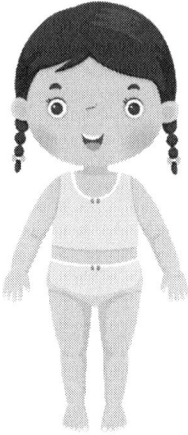

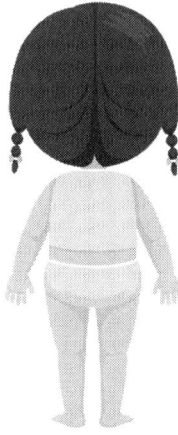

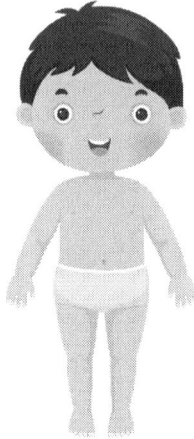

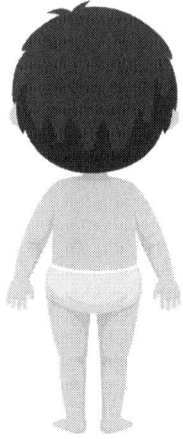

Notes

	Time	Blood Sugar	Carbs	Insulin	Notes
Breakfast					
Snack					
Lunch					
Snack					
Dinner					
Bedtime					
Night					

Shot Location

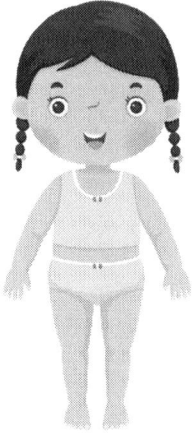

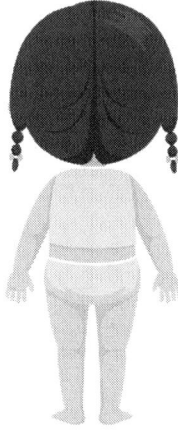

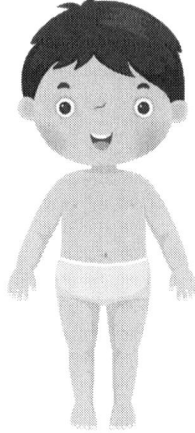

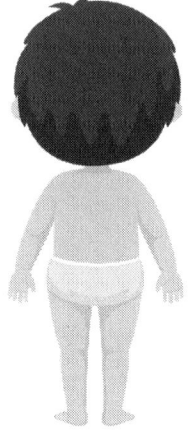

Notes

	Time	Blood Sugar	Carbs	Insulin	Notes
Breakfast					
Snack					
Lunch					
Snack					
Dinner					
Bedtime					
Night					

Shot Location

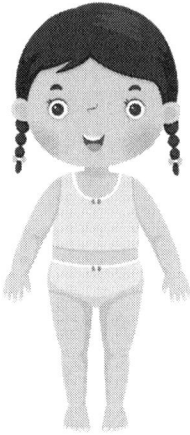

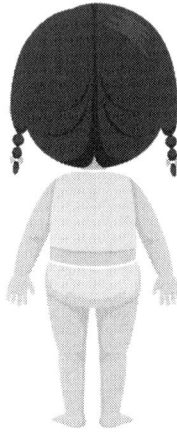

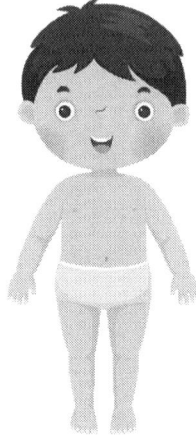

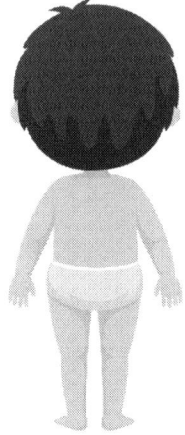

Notes

	Time	Blood Sugar	Carbs	Insulin	Notes
Breakfast					
Snack					
Lunch					
Snack					
Dinner					
Bedtime					
Night					

Shot Location

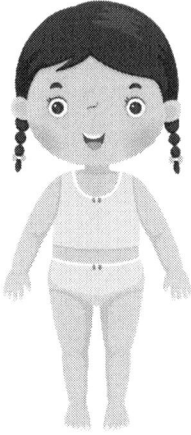

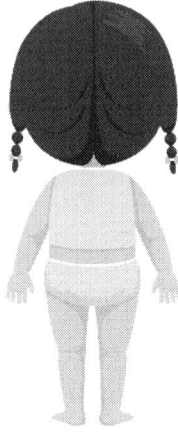

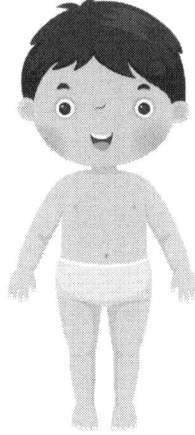

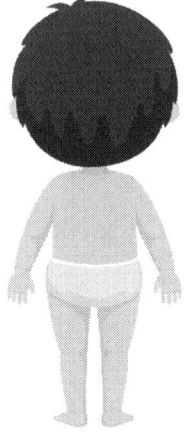

Notes

	Time	Blood Sugar	Carbs	Insulin	Notes
Breakfast					
Snack					
Lunch					
Snack					
Dinner					
Bedtime					
Night					

Shot Location

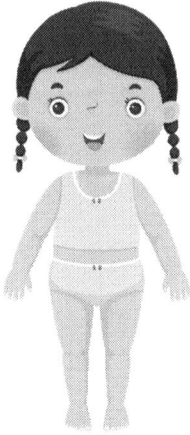

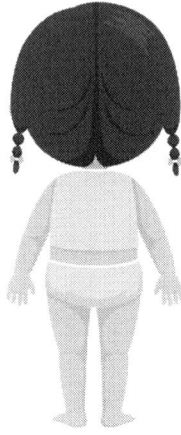

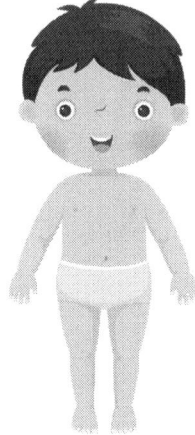

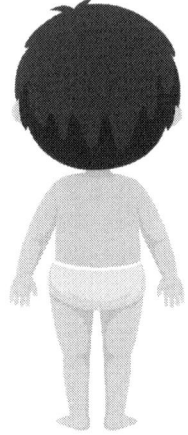

Notes

	Time	Blood Sugar	Carbs	Insulin	Notes
Breakfast					
Snack					
Lunch					
Snack					
Dinner					
Bedtime					
Night					

Shot Location

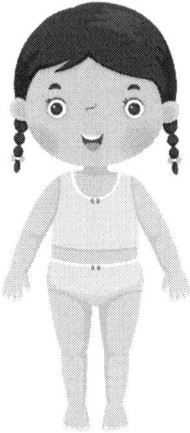

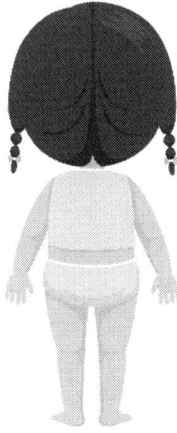

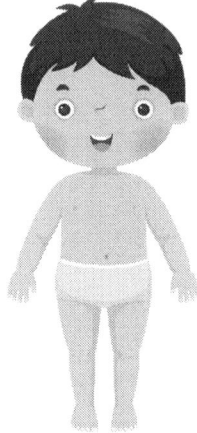

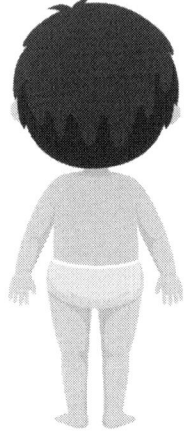

Notes

	Time	Blood Sugar	Carbs	Insulin	Notes
Breakfast					
Snack					
Lunch					
Snack					
Dinner					
Bedtime					
Night					

Shot Location

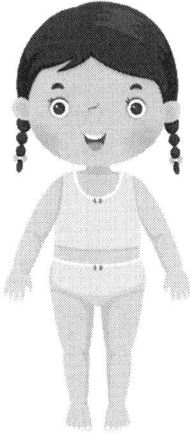

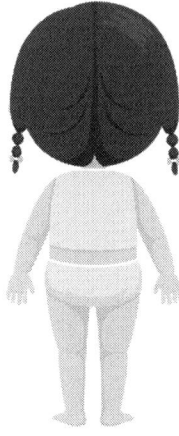

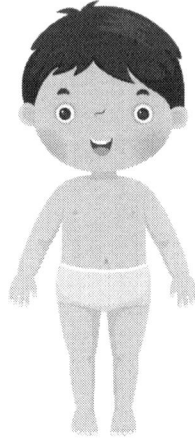

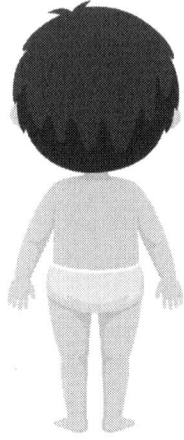

Notes

	Time	Blood Sugar	Carbs	Insulin	Notes
Breakfast					
Snack					
Lunch					
Snack					
Dinner					
Bedtime					
Night					

Shot Location

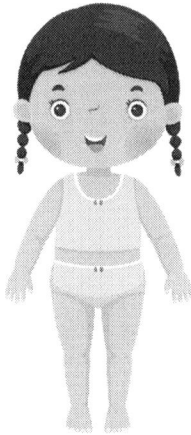

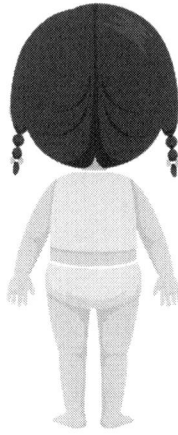

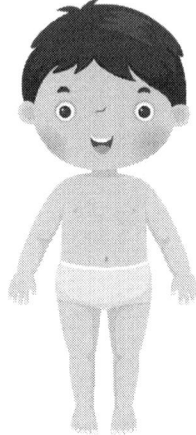

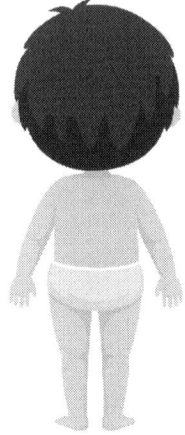

Notes

	Time	Blood Sugar	Carbs	Insulin	Notes
Breakfast					
Snack					
Lunch					
Snack					
Dinner					
Bedtime					
Night					

Shot Location

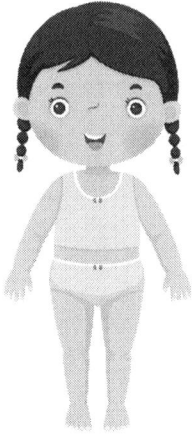

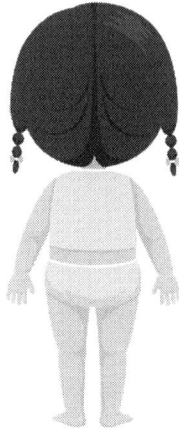

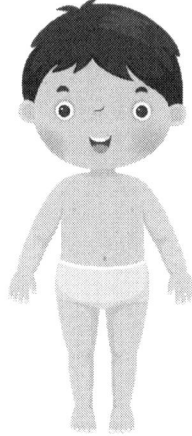

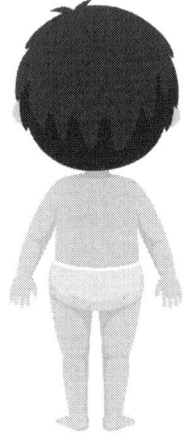

Notes

	Time	Blood Sugar	Carbs	Insulin	Notes
Breakfast					
Snack					
Lunch					
Snack					
Dinner					
Bedtime					
Night					

Shot Location

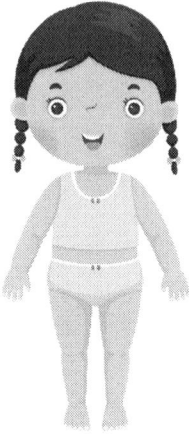

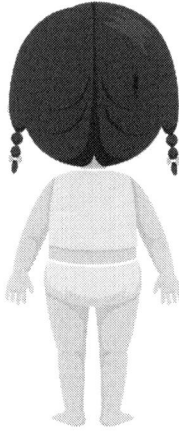

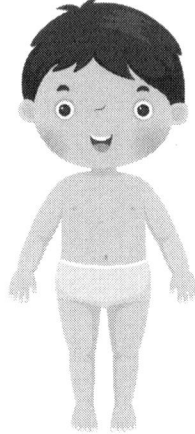

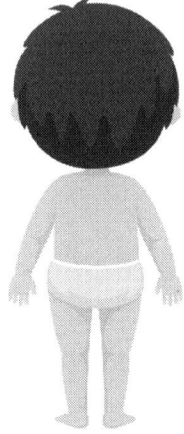

Notes

	Time	Blood Sugar	Carbs	Insulin	Notes
Breakfast					
Snack					
Lunch					
Snack					
Dinner					
Bedtime					
Night					

Shot Location

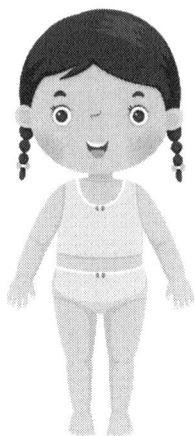

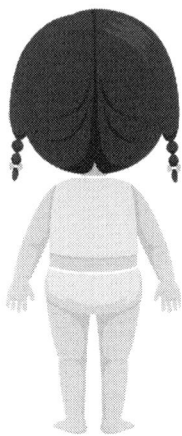

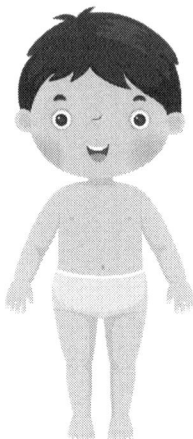

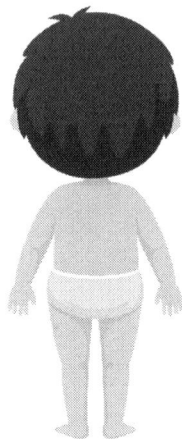

Notes

	Time	Blood Sugar	Carbs	Insulin	Notes
Breakfast					
Snack					
Lunch					
Snack					
Dinner					
Bedtime					
Night					

Shot Location

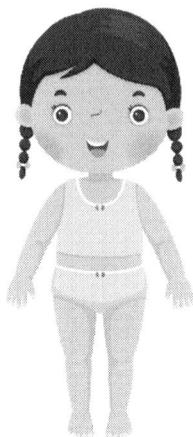

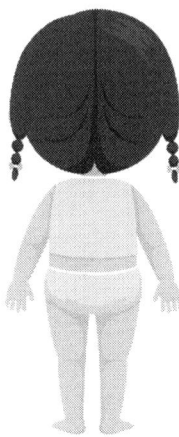

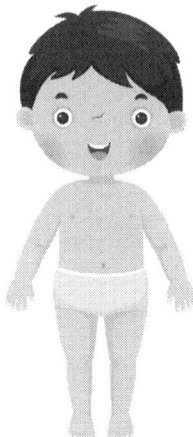

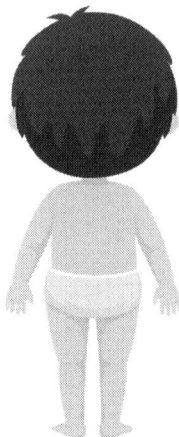

Notes

	Time	Blood Sugar	Carbs	Insulin	Notes
Breakfast					
Snack					
Lunch					
Snack					
Dinner					
Bedtime					
Night					

Shot Location

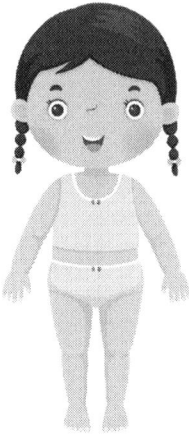

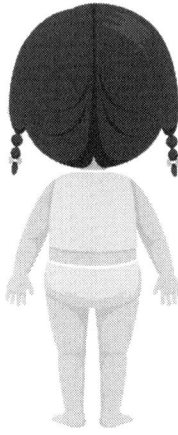

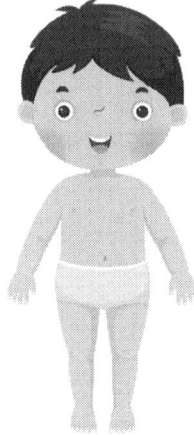

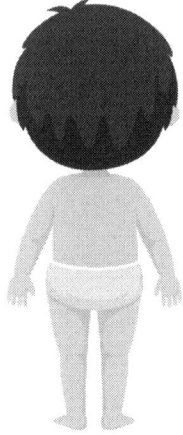

Notes

	Time	Blood Sugar	Carbs	Insulin	Notes
Breakfast					
Snack					
Lunch					
Snack					
Dinner					
Bedtime					
Night					

Shot Location

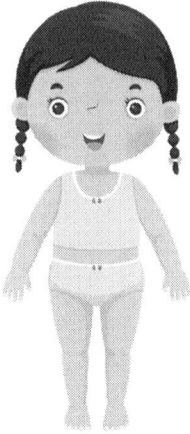

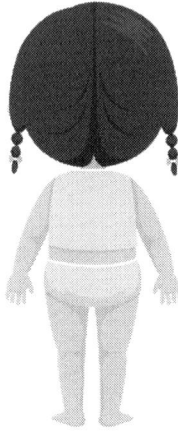

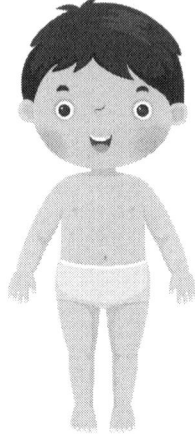

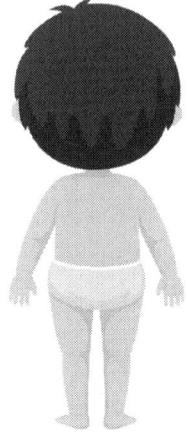

Notes

	Time	Blood Sugar	Carbs	Insulin	Notes
Breakfast					
Snack					
Lunch					
Snack					
Dinner					
Bedtime					
Night					

Shot Location

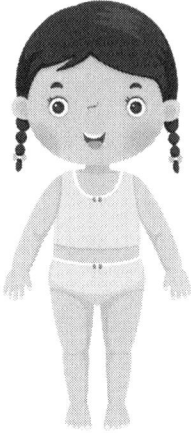

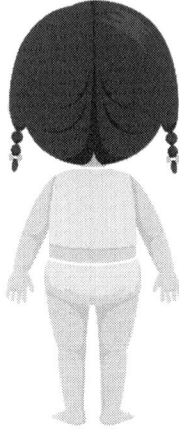

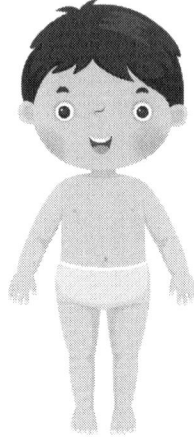

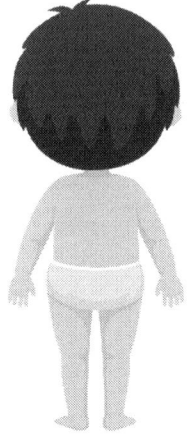

Notes

	Time	Blood Sugar	Carbs	Insulin	Notes
Breakfast					
Snack					
Lunch					
Snack					
Dinner					
Bedtime					
Night					

Made in the USA
Las Vegas, NV
23 September 2022